95 Tips to Win the Mental Game of Running

Strategies for Overcoming Mental Blocks and Becoming the Best Runner Possible

By Amber Hadigan

Hadigan, Amber
95 Tips to Win the Mental Game of Running: Strategies for Overcoming Mental Blocks and Becoming the Best Runner Possible / Amber Hadigan – 1st Ed.

ISBN-10: 1530420083
ISBN-13: 978-1530420087

This book is dedicated to all my running friends. Just by putting on your shoes, you have inspired me, motivated me, and taught me what it takes to be a great runner. Thank you for running.

Table of Contents

Preface

As a struggling runner, there are days when lacing up my shoes and getting outside seems almost impossible. I am not fast, I am not light, I do not have a typical runner's body, and running can sometimes be a very difficult task for me. I spent a long time trying to figure out ways to motivate me in those moments where running seemed too difficult to do. I learned everything I could. I read every book on running I could get my hands on. I asked friends and in running groups on Facebook what they do to inspire themselves, even when the task of running seemed monumental. When I start something, I learn everything I can. I consult many different sources for inspiration and try to become an expert. When I started running, it was no different. I wanted to have all the tips, tricks, and tools at my fingertips to make it easier, both physically and mentally. I took notes and kept track of what worked for me and what didn't. I revised my list, making sure it made sense to me. I also tracked things that worked for others, but not necessarily for myself.

My obsessive note-taking, tracking, and experimenting has made me a better runner. It has not necessarily made me faster, but it has made me more consistent. I went from struggling while running 3 days per week, for just a few miles each run, to being able to train for a marathon five days a week, with my short runs being at least 5 miles and my long runs hitting a maximum of twenty miles.

This book is the accumulation of the results of this obsessive investigating and tracking. My desire is to save you the work that I went through of coming up with different ways to motivate yourself. I hope that you find the techniques and tricks in this book helpful to get you out the door and make running a priority in your life.

About the Author

Amber Hadigan has her Master's Degree in Transpersonal Psychology from Sophia University. She is a singer/songwriter, writer, and marathon runner. She has been writing poetry and nonfiction for as long as she can remember.

Introduction

It has been said that 90 percent of running is a mental game. After you have trained your body to handle the physical demands of running, most people are under the mistaken impression that running should be easy to do. But the truth is, although the physical act of running isn't too difficult once you are in shape, the mental aspects of running can be a much harder thing to conquer. Runners need to train their brains to keep moving long after they wish to give up. It is true that your mind will want to quit long before your body actually needs to, so it is important to teach the mind how to keep going when it gets tougher. Therefore, all runners need to train their brain as much, if not more so, than their bodies.

I wrote this book with the hope that you would learn many different tips and tricks you can try to improve the mental game of running. When your mind is ready to quit, you need to convince it to keep going. After all, you can run far longer than your legs wish to admit. You can work on training your mind, before the run, while you are in the middle of the run and possibly struggling, and after you have finished. By doing so, you will improve your mental game and make running easier and more enjoyable. Remember, your body can go far longer than you give it credit for, and if you can conquer your mind, you can improve your running and your life.

This book is separated sections based on when to do each exercise: things to do between runs, while preparing for a run, mental games to keep going during a run, and what to do after a run is completed. By having a routine for all the times of your day that relate to your running, you will become a more successful runner. These things do not take up much time, but they will really help you win the mental game of running. Although you are not running all the time, whenever you think of running, you can use one of these quick strategies to improve your run. And, during your run, when you think you cannot go on, you can use one of these techniques to keep going, improve your performance, and even feel better physically and mentally.

Not all of these tips will work for everyone. In fact, some of them may even be the exact opposite of another one. This is because not every tip will work for everyone, and not every tip will work every day. I have found that what works for me on Monday may not work on Wednesday. Depending on my state of mind and my physical needs, opposite tricks may work on different days. For example, one day I find that tuning out and finding distractions will work on a run, while on another day, I need to pay attention to what is happening with my body. The mind is a fickle thing, and needs to be convinced, over and over, to do what you want it to do. So, try them all. Give them a go, and if it doesn't work one day, it may work the next. Soon, you will find the keys that make your running more successful and even a little easier. The key is to figure out what works for you when and to use those techniques consistently so that your mind and body become more in sync. By finding the best ones, you will become a better runner.

Who am I to write this book? Frankly, I'm not fast. I'm not great. But I persevere. In the time I have been running, I went from not being able to go more than thirty seconds at a time to running marathons. At first, I couldn't get out the door for more than two minutes before feeling like I was going to die. Now I go for long runs of twenty miles. And I'm a normal person. I'm 41 years old, I work, have a home and husband, and plenty of outside obligations. So, basically, I am like you. I work hard, play hard, and want to improve myself, both on and off the trail. And I've used these tricks and techniques to improve my running ability. I've also gleaned tricks from my running friends who, like you, are just trying to improve themselves. The ideas in this book come from the contributions of many runners who have dug deep and succeeded at winning the mental game of running.

So happy running and good luck! We all could use it from time to time.

What to Do In Between Runs

There are many things you can do throughout your day to prepare your mind for running. In fact, many of these tips have been used in a variety of settings to make improvements in different areas of your life, which means that they could help with other things going on for you, not just running. When you become a runner, running will occupy your mind throughout the day, not just when you are on the trails. Using these suggestions, you can harness your wandering thoughts to improve your running game. Check out these tips to improve your running when you are not running. Figure out which ones work best for you and use them consistently. They won't take much time out of your day, but they will help you see big improvements when you do lace up your shoes. To become a better runner, training your mind to be positive away from your training will make it easier when it is time to put on your shoes.

1. Buy *The Little Engine That Could*: Remember this book from your childhood? Most of us had it read to us long before we were able to read it ourselves. It's about the little train engine that was trying to push a big train up the hill. It seemed an impossible task, yet the engine kept repeating "I think I can, I think I can." Watty Piper, the author, sure knew what he was talking about! Well, running works exactly the same way. Read this book to remind yourself of this mantra

and the idea that belief can conquer almost anything. "I think I can" became a mantra for me while hill training a few weeks ago, and since then I have kept a copy of this little volume on my desk to remind me that I can do anything that I put my mind to. You, too, can benefit from repeating these words, both during your run and when you are thinking about running.

2. Visualization: One of the most utilized techniques in the world for improved performance in almost any field is visualization. When you visualize something, you imagine in your mind's eye what will happen when you do that activity. For example, if you imagine every step of a goal race in your mind, you will train your mind to complete it in a similar way. Close your eyes and see yourself running strong, fast, and comfortable. Imagine each step you take and how good it feels. Imagine all your movements. Think about proper form, calm, unlabored breathing, and even the smile on your face. Do this for five minutes every day.

One of the most accomplished athletes in the world that makes use of regular visualization is Michael Phelps, winner of 22 Olympic medals. He uses his time outside the pool to imagine in his mind's eye every move of his swim, from how he jumps in (perfectly), to a perfect kick off the wall, and how his strokes will be. He envisions every step of a race and imagines himself swimming perfectly, fluidly, and feels it in his body when he sees it in his mind.

It has been shown that mental training such as this helps the body perform better, and can even be as good as physical training itself. Imagine your stride, running with perfect form, and how you will conquer that hill. Although it won't replace your physical training, it is a great adjunct to the physical work.

Studies have even shown that visualization helps to train your mind and body to perform better when you are engaging in the activity you visualize. Therefore, if you see yourself as strong and comfortable in your mind, you will feel more like that when you really are running. Just make sure that you can see every aspect. Visualization is a directed goal, not just a day dream. Make sure that you use your visualization as a training tool, not just a fantasy.

3. Find a hero: Everyone needs someone to look up to for motivation. In running, I have a couple heroes. First is Meb, the only person to win the Boston Marathon (2014), the New York Marathon (2009), and an Olympic medal in the marathon (2004). Although I will never be as fast as Meb, I find him a down-to-earth and inspiring athlete that anyone can look up to. My other running hero is a friend of mine. She is like me: in her 40s, has a real life outside of running, and makes the

time to train for marathons. She has never won a medal or qualified for Boston, but when I see her post on Facebook, it reminds me that I can do this too. When I think of these two people and what they do day in and day out, I am motivated to continue my own running journey. I am particularly inspired by people who are like me that still make time to train.

You may not even have to know your running hero. I see one particular person on a path I use frequently. Almost every time I am out, I see her running. She is overweight, looks like she is struggling, yet she never gives up. She has also inspired me. I've nodded and said good morning, though I don't even know her name. She is one of my heroes.

By finding your own running hero, you will have someone to turn to when you feel discouraged. If it is someone famous, you can think of what they go through to run as a career. If it is a friend, you can even call them when you're feeling low and maybe go for a run together. Just knowing there are people out there doing the same thing you are and working through the same problems can make it easier to get out there every day. Other runners are very inspiring.

4. Set a goal: Having a goal gives you a reason to run, especially when you're feeling discouraged. Many people start running to lose weight or get in shape, but an ambiguous goal makes it difficult to get motivated. Instead, make sure your goal is measurable. For example, if you want to lose weight, set a small weight goal, such as ten pounds. That gives you something to work for and a way to measure your success.

Runners, however, often find a running goal more motivating. You could sign up for a target race for a new distance, race for a new PR, set a time goal (such as, I want to run a ten minute mile), or a number of days you will run a week (I will run 30 minutes a day four days per week). A quantifiable goal is the easiest to stick to because you can easily measure your progress. And you'll feel great about yourself when you achieve your particular goal.

The important thing when setting a goal is to keep it challenging but attainable. If it's too easy to achieve, there is nothing to work for. On the other hand, if you can't run more than a minute at a time, it might be too soon to sign up for a marathon. If the goal is too hard, most people give up in frustration before really beginning to do the work.

5. Evaluate your goals and pay attention to your training: Make sure that your goals, once you have them, are reasonable. For example, it makes no sense to set a goal of running 50 miles per week if you are just starting. By setting a goal that is unattainable right now, you'll actually discourage your running and give up quickly. This is a dramatic example, but it personifies the need to evaluate what you are doing.

Take the example of running 30 minutes per day, four days per week. Let's say, after running three or four weeks, you are finding that you are struggling to get that fourth day in. This could be for any number of reasons, such as having the time to run or not be giving your body enough time between runs to recover (since you may just be starting out). There is no shame in reevaluating your goals and cutting back to three days per week. After you have made this goal a habit, you can reevaluate again and see if you can go back up to four days, or if you want to run 45 minutes instead of 30. As your running improves, after you suffer an injury, or your scheduling commitments change, you may have to reevaluate what you are doing to match up with your life. Your goals should be challenging, but not impossible for you to meet.

Once you achieve a goal, set a new one quickly. I know that I lose focus between training cycles if I don't set a new goal. Make sure you have something up your sleeve.

6. Don't compare yourself to others: We all make this mistake. Everyone looks at the person next to them to see how they measure up. Whether you run in a group and compare yourself to a running partner or you compare yourself to the person you end up in line with at a race, you want something to measure yourself by. You could even be comparing yourself to some unknown runner that you seed posting in a Facebook running group! However, comparing yourself to other runners is like comparing apples and oranges.

I normally train by myself, but while training for a half marathon in my town, I trained with a group raising money for the SPCA. One woman I ran with had a Boston Qualifying time, while I struggled to keep up an 11 minute pace over long runs. At times, I became frustrated when I ran with her, such as when I saw her take off or I tried to keep up with her insane pace. But, when I sat down to think about it, there were several things going on. First, she was younger than me. She was also skinnier (less weight to carry down the trail makes for a faster runner), and she had been running much longer than I had. If I allowed myself to get upset or discouraged because she could run faster and better than I, I never would have trained again.

Instead, the only person I choose to compare myself to is the person I was before. Two years ago, I couldn't run three miles without walking. I was overweight and got winded walking up a flight of stairs. Now, I can run a half marathon without a break, and have completed two full marathons (with walk breaks). Future goals include running an entire marathon and setting new PRs. All I can do is look at how far I have come and be proud of my efforts.

If I compare myself to anyone else, I will only see failure. If I compare myself to who I was yesterday, I am a winner!

7.   Sign up for a race: Most runners use races as a goal. When you run, whether it be by yourself or with a group, it just doesn't compare to the feeling of running a race. Hundreds or even thousands of people are around you, all with the same goal, water stops, cool t-shirts, possibly a medal at the end, and a specific date all make a race a common goal many runners strive for. They are fun, they give you something to look forward to, and you can surround yourself with like

minds who also have been training hard. Races are booming, and there are plenty in almost any area, from a one mile sprint to a marathon and even larger, such as 50 mile ultras! So there is a race for everyone out there.

Just make sure to give yourself enough time to train. If you've been running for a while, you can probably do a 5K on short notice, but longer races do require a little bit of time to prepare for. If you are a genuine beginner, it could take eight weeks or more to train for a 5K, which is the length of most training plans. For a marathon, it could be 16 weeks or more, depending on your fitness level.

8.   Surround yourself with people who motivate you: Studies have shown that we are a combination of the five people we spend the most time with. This means that we tend to pick up the habits of the people we are closest to. So, if you hang out with people who are sedentary and don't exercise, you are more likely to do the same. Therefore, if you are just starting to run, or are looking for some motivation, find yourself runners to spend time with. Check your area for a local running store, which is likely to sponsor group runs or training runs. Look for a local Road Runners club, who may host trainings, races, and other activities. You can even look for

runners on the Meetup website, where people put ads looking for people with like interests (it's not a hook-up site), including exercise partners. Many areas also sponsor beginner's running classes, where they help a group of people just starting to run train for and run a 5K. Contact local running stores, a running group, or outdoor groups to see if someone has formed such a class. You will be motivated by spending time with people who talk about running and who you could even run with.

9. Keep a list of why you run: What motivated you to start running? Write those reasons down. Keep this list handy, so if you need any motivation to get out or you are having a bad day, you can look at it and remind yourself of your goals, your desires, and why you started in the first place. You don't want to forget these reasons.

My list includes such things as:
To lose weight
To stay sane
To feel like I accomplished something
To get outside
To have fun
To earn cool t-shirts and medals

Different goals motivate me on different days. It helps to have several reasons.

10. Get a new piece of gear: Everyone likes cool stuff. Whether it be a GPS watch so you can track all your stats, a new pair of shoes, a beautiful training journal to keep track of your progress, or an awesome, colorful new pair of shorts, a new piece of gear is always a great way to motivate yourself to hit the pavement. Me, I love new shoes and funky clothes, those that make me stand out when I cross the finish line and even get the announcer to comment on my outfit (it's happened a couple times). If you are a little bored with your training, getting yourself something new can get you back in the game.

11. Hang out at the running store: Spend some time getting to know the people that work there. Oftentimes, you will interact directly with the manager or owner. You will meet other runners, learn about local training groups and races, and just get that good vibe. Some running stores even have seminars sponsored by either the store or companies that make running gear. If you have one close to you, check it out

regularly. You'll connect with awesome people, learn a thing or two about your hobby, and get inspired.

12. Keep a training log: It's important to keep track of your running. Especially when starting out, you want to know what you are running, how long, and what your goals are. This gives you the ability to go back and see how much you have improved. It can also help you pinpoint the reasons you may be struggling. If you're just starting and you can only run two minutes at a time, then you go back and look at your log later, you can see the progress you have made. Being able to track your progress is a great motivator. You know that you are making improvements over time.

There are many ways to keep a running log. Paper journals, printed by many different companies, are great, as you can record whatever you want, including distance, time, where you ran, notes on how you felt, and even keep track of the weather. Other options include an app on your phone or tablet, or online recorders such as Map My Run, Runkeeper, or Garmin Connect, if you have one of their GPS devices. I like to use a combination of an app called Runner's Log and a physical, handwritten journal because I have a beautiful, leather-bound journal. The app keeps track of my numbers easily, such as miles run in a week and month and how many miles are on each pair of shoes. I keep a paper log because I love writing and the feel of the paper under my fingers. Between the two, everything gets recorded.

13. Reward yourself: Almost everyone is willing to keep going if there is something worthwhile at the end. It could be a small reward to get through a run, or a larger one when you complete a training and race cycle. After training for my first half marathon, I bought myself a new running outfit. After a long run when I have difficulty, I reward myself with a new book or magazine I have been wanting. It gives me an incentive to keep going when things get tough. If I don't finish, I don't get the reward.

Pick out something that you want, but try not to make it food. Especially if you are trying to lose weight, a food reward may actually move to sabotage your efforts. But just about anything else is fair game.

14. Read motivational stories: I love books on running. There seems to be two types: the first are training books, which give you recommendations for how to train, what to eat, and other similar advice. The other type of book are those with

motivational stories of other runners. These are my absolute favorite. When I read a story about a runner who has overcome something, it really makes me want to put on my shoes and head out the door. I have several of these books, and have been known to read and reread them when I hit a slump. One good story before bed is enough to get me up early in the morning for my run.

Some books that have been particularly motivating for me include:

Going Long: Legends, Oddballs, Comebacks, and Adventurers, edited by the Editors of Runner's world and David Willey

Marathon Woman by Kathrine Switzer

Marathon Man by Bill Rodgers and Matthew Shepatin

Running & Being: The Total Experience by George Sheehan

The Terrible and Wonderful Reasons Why I Run Long Distances by The Oatmeal (Matthew Inman)

Running With the Mind of Meditation by Sakyong Mipham

This list will get you started. Check out your local bookstore or library for many more titles. Many websites also list some of the best running books available. Check them out.

15. Pay yourself: Every time you go for a run, put a dollar (or five) in a jar. Use this money to buy that new piece of gear that you had your eye on or even pay for a run-cation, where you travel somewhere you've always wanted to go to run a race. The more you run, the faster you will earn that one expensive piece that you have been craving. A new jacket, GPS watch, or a trip can then be earned, and trying to get there will motivate you to get out the door.

16. Find a coach: Although there are plenty of books, magazines, and websites on running, telling us how to train, what to eat, and when to taper, sometimes that just doesn't seem to be enough. At this point, many people go on to hire a running coach. The joys of utilizing a coach include getting customized training plans and having someone to be accountable to. When you are paying someone to tell you when and how to run, you are more likely to do it, especially when you have to report back on a daily or weekly basis. There may be a coach in your area, or you can find a coach online.

Plus, a coach can be your best cheerleader. Having someone there to encourage you, to keep you motivated, and to figure out how to get you moving and how you will improve, is an awesome thing. Plus, you will love having someone answer your questions, keep you upbeat, and offer you advice when you need it most. Most runners find paying a coach a worthwhile investment.

17. Use motivational quotes: I'm a sucker for Facebook. I belong to several running groups and have liked several running pages for one reason: seeing running memes with motivational quotes at the start of the day really inspires me. Whether talking about overcoming hardship, inspiring you with the beauty of nature, or just reminding yourself of your goals, motivational quotes can do this. I have been known to print them up and put them on my wall, use them as background on my iPad and laptop, and even share them on my wall on Facebook to back to them when I need a lift. They have also become mantras during a run when I need to inspire myself. When you need a little nudge out the door, just google "running memes" for a little bit of inspiration.

18. Try a runner's streak: The idea behind a running streak is to run at least a mile every day for a certain amount of time. I first saw this idea in *Runner's World Magazine*, where they do streaks twice a year, one from Memorial Day to the Fourth of July, and the other from Thanksgiving to New Years. They have chosen these times because they are usually dead times in someone's training, after the spring or the fall race season, when people tend to slack. They even host a Facebook page so streakers can connect with each other and stay motivated during their streak.

Although *Runner's World* hosts streaks twice a year, you can choose to start your own streak any time you want. Pick a day to start, and on the days you are supposed to rest during your training, you run one easy mile. Don't go hard out and don't push the pace. Run a single nice, easy mile. It's a reason to put your shoes on every day and keeps you going. Some people enjoy doing small streaks (I like to do them about 45 days at a time), and there are others who take their streaking to whole new levels. Some people have streaks going for months and years. The longest documented streaker ran every day for 45 years before giving it up! You don't have to keep it up for years, but running a streak, even for a month, can get your mojo flowing again.

19. Schedule your run: Pull out your calendar and make a date with yourself to run. Make an appointment that cannot be broken. Don't schedule anything else during that time. Your run is a commitment you make with yourself, and when you schedule it, it makes it much easier to get out there. It is a promise, and as your mother said, you should never break a promise. I like to do this on a weekly basis, when I plan my week on Sunday night. A date with yourself should be just as important as a date with a business colleague.

20. Try the Zombies run! App: Zombies Run! is an app for your smartphone that will motivate you during a workout. When you turn on the app, it gives you a mission. During your workout, when the app says you are being chased by zombies, you have to speed up to avoid them. If you don't, you will get eaten and you will fail your mission. Many people find the app inspiring and fun. Download it and give it a try. Maybe you could save the world!

21. Challenge friends on Map My Run: Map My Run is another app that you can download to your phone, which uses a GPS tracker to keep track of your miles, speed, and distance. You can also friend others on the app and share

data. Your friends can see what you do, and you can see their runs. I have a friend who swears by this app, and he told me that it encourages him to go out and get more miles. If he ran three miles in the morning, but then a friend ran five, he may be tempted to go out and do two more so that person doesn't get ahead of him. If competition spurs you, this may be a great way to stay motivated by your friends.

22. Use doubters as fuel: Everyone has someone tell them they can't do something. Some people will start doubting your ability to run a race. You may have heard things such as "You'll never be able to run a 5K, or a marathon." Some people believe it when people tell them this and give up. However, turn it around. Use their doubt to fuel your motivation.

While watching the Boston Marathon in 2015, I was curious, so looked up the Boston qualifying time for my age and gender. It was 3:45. Now, I had only run one marathon in my life to that point, and it was 5:46. Therefore, for me to qualify for Boston, I would need to drop my marathon time by over two hours! When I told my husband what my BQ time would be, he looked at me and said, "You'll never do it," and turned back to whatever he was doing. Since he said that, I have been training for another marathon. It may take years for me to get to the point that I can qualify, but his doubt about my ability to improve enough to BQ lingers in the back of my mind. I would love to prove him wrong. This keeps me motivated through marathon training and may even keep me running marathons for years to come!

23. Bling: It always feels good to have something to show off your running accomplishments. Many runners sign up for races in order to get bling, specifically medals and other goodies. I recently ran The Boilermaker, a 15K held every year in Utica, New York. A woman I spoke to said it was her twelfth one, and she does it for the pint glasses they give to every registered runner. I, personally, love getting race T-shirts. Others love medals and take great pride in showing them off on Facebook and making displays for them in their home. Getting bling motivates many people when other things do not.

If you want bling, make sure to check out what a race offers you when you sign up. Most races will specify if you get a t-shirt, a medal, or anything else. Larger races also may have things for sale that relate to the race. I love to buy the baseball cap for races I run, if they have one. Usually races that are a half marathon or longer offer better bling than shorter races.

24. Sign up for a crazy race: Color runs, tough mudders, and inflatable obstacle races are all very popular. It could be that you are bored with a traditional race and want something different or that you are looking for the challenge an obstacle race provides, allowing you to mix up your training. Signing up for one of these new types of races can reignite your desire to run. Plus, if you are running an obstacle course, it will spur you on to cross train and try something new, such as strength training. And getting stronger will improve your running.

25. Visualize obstacles and how to overcome them: If there is a specific obstacle that thwarts your running, use some visualization time to imagine how you will overcome that obstacle. It plants the seed in your mind so that, when you do have a problem, your brain has already been trained on a solution.

Again, using visualization is a time-tested strategy for athletes of all kinds. If you struggle with something specific, you can use visualization to overcome this obstacle in your mind. This will reinforce a positive approach when you actually encounter this issue during your run. For example, my biggest running problem is getting tired half-way through my long runs and walking, rather than keeping myself moving. So I have incorporated visualization in my training. I imagine what I feel like when I get tired and want to walk, and I see myself running through the fatigue. I imagine how that will feel. There have been times when I have done so, so I understand what it feels like to do it. I remind myself during the visualization that my body does recover and can even feel good, if I just keep going at the point of lowest fatigue. Through this, I plant the idea of forward running in my mind, even when tired. That way, when I encounter this problem in real life, this message will already be there, making it harder to just give up.

You can use this same visualization strategy for any issue you may have during your run. If you can see yourself overcoming the difficulty, you can do it in real life.

26. Plan a race-cation: This works especially well if you live in a cold climate in the winter or a really hot climate in the summer. Pick a warm climate to go to in January, or a cooler place to run in August. Sign up for a race at that location. It gives you the motivation to train because you don't want to pay a great deal of money to run a race, travel, and get a

hotel room, and not be ready for it. Plus, it gives you the opportunity to have a good time after the race. Make it a real vacation and stay, sightsee, and try some new restaurants. But plan the race for early in your trip. That way, you can race, and then enjoy yourself without the worry of your venture hanging over your head.

27. Take a rest day: It may sound counterintuitive, but rest is a necessity for running. Your body needs time to repair itself from the trauma running puts it through. Don't run seven days a week (unless you are on a streak, see above). If your body is telling you to rest, it's good to listen to it. It prevents injuries and makes your next run even better. Contrary to popular belief, there is no shame in needing a rest, and you will even feel better the next day!

28. Cut back your mileage for one week every month: This Is a necessity, especially if you rack up a lot of miles. For example, most marathon and half marathon training plans cut back mileage every three or four week. So, if you do three 15-20 mile long runs, the fourth week will cut back that long run to eight or ten miles. This helps your body and mind have the chance to recover. If you push yourself too hard without giving both your body and your mind a chance to recover, you

may just teach yourself to hate your run, which usually results in quitting. Cutting back the mileage will give yourself a break and hopefully reignite your passion for running because it doesn't have to be such a grind.

29. Make several goals for a race or a run: Most people set one single goal for a race, and, if they don't make that goal, they then see the race as a failure. However, most expert coaches suggest setting up as many as three goals for a single race: a main goal, a second goal, and a third goal. For example, when I ran my first marathon, my first goal was to run it in under 5:30, my second goal was to not walk, and my third goal was to finish (it was my first marathon, after all). When it became clear 5:30 was out of the question because I had walked, I still felt proud of the accomplishment because I made at least one of my goals.

Your main goal will be the best possible scenario. It should be difficult, but not impossible, to complete. If you make this goal, you will be on cloud nine. Your secondary goal will be slightly easier to make, but still difficult. The third goal will be easier still, but it will still be an accomplishment to do. In my example, when I finished the marathon in 5:46, I was still very happy because I had finished before being swept, as the course had a 6 hour time limit. Although I didn't make my first two goals, I was still satisfied with my performance. MY third goal is usually the least I will be happy with, the second goal will be a little harder, and the first will be my ideal, perfect race scenario (they do happen!).

30. Have a cheerleader: It's always helpful to have someone on your side, whether it be another runner or someone in your life to keep you going. My husband does that for me. Although he isn't a runner, he always asks me about my runs, makes sure I get out the door, and comes to some of my races to be there for me. It always keeps me going to know that someone is keeping an eye on my progress and cheering me on for the small wins. No matter who it is, whether it be a significant other, a friend, or someone on Facebook that you may not have even met except in a virtual running group, knowing that someone is cheering you on and thinking about your efforts really helps to keep you in lIne.

31. Work on your attitude: Sometimes my running attitude sucks. I'll tell myself that my mind just isn't into it and use it as an excuse to cut a workout short or to walk when I can still run. I set myself up for failure when I expect a run to be bad. Instead, if I catch myself having these negative thoughts and

replace them with something more positive, my runs go easier. A negative attitude or mindset will affect how you run. I will often think something like, "I don't want to do this anymore." When this happens, I consciously change my mindset and replace that thought with a more positive one, such as, "I am strong." Changing my mind mid-run always makes the run a little easier. Sometimes an attitude adjustment is a necessity.

This isn't just important in the middle of a run. It is also a necessity when you think about running during your day. Sometimes you may catch yourself thinking about how you don't want to run when you get home, or dreading a long run the next day. When you think those negative thoughts, it is up to you to catch yourself and replace them. For example, if you are dreading running 20 miles tomorrow (or five, or whatever), remind yourself that you are strong and capable of conquering the miles. Change the negative thought to a positive one. Find a reason to look forward to your long run.

32. Find a friend: Training with another person gives you two things: moral support and someone to be accountable to. If you are running with someone else, you now have someone who is holding you accountable for your run. It's harder to

back out of a run when someone is waiting for you. Although I usually run alone, I have found that those days that I run with someone else gives my run a different feel. Matching paces doesn't seem so hard, conversation keeps things interesting, and the time passes much faster. Although I usually love my solitude when I run, those times that I have a companion are to be remembered.

33. Make a running creed: A motto, creed, or mantra will keep you going. Repeat it in your mind when you run, when you are preparing to run, and whenever you think about running. Come up with the reason you run, what you hope to get out of it, and make a one-line phrase. Post it on your computer, in the bathroom, and in your car. It'll remind you why you are doing this. If you aren't sure what to use, search the Internet for running memes. There are plenty of great creeds and mantras on the Internet. When you find one that inspires you, print it out and hold it close to your heart. Write it down and put it in places that will remind you of your goals. This way, you will keep your training goals in the forefront of your mind, even when you aren't training.

34. Get the App Pact: Pact is an app that you download and make a commitment to working out and eating right. You

choose your goals that you want to achieve and you make a promise to pay a certain amount of money if you do not reach these goals. You get to decide what you will pay if you do not complete them. Then the app tracks your progress. If you complete your run as you committed to, you get paid by others. If you do not complete it, you pay the amount specified when you signed up. Financial motivation is a very powerful one!

35. Variety is the spice of life: Do something different. Try a new route, run with others if you normally run alone, or run alone if you run with a group. Have you always run on the road? Try a trail. Try a track workout. Make a new running playlist or go without music. Doing the same thing day after day gets boring and makes it less likely for you to keep going. When you start to get bored, do something, anything, to mix up your run.

By using small pockets of time when you are not running to train your mind, you will make it easier when you are out on the road. Find a few minutes during each day to do this, and you will see improvements on the run. The next chapter will give you ideas for how to prepare your mind for when you are preparing to hit the trail or the pavement.

Preparing for a run

The time you spend preparing for your run is important to how you mentally approach your run. The time you spend physically getting ready for a run, such as eating a snack, getting dressed, and lacing your shoes properly, can also be used to help prepare your mind. You can use the time to get in the right mindset, visualize your run, and repeat mantras, among other exercises. When you do these things, you set the stage for a good, solid, productive outing. Failure to prepare mentally can make the run more difficult. Here are some great ways to prepare for your run in the time immediately before you head out the door. Try some of these activities to improve your mental preparation when you are getting ready to go run.

1. Routine: Have a pre-run routine that you follow every time. Do the same things before every race and every workout. This makes it easier to get you in the right mindset. Doing the same thing in the same order every time sets the stage for a good run and prepares your mind for the work that is to come. I like to lay out my clothes, have a pre-run fuel up, go to the bathroom (about five times), and get dressed. I always make sure that I have everything I need, including fluids, my house key, phone, and iPod. Especially when I am driving for a run or preparing for a race, doing the same

routine each time helps me make sure that I don't forget anything and that I am mentally prepared to run.

2. Commit publicly: It helps to tell people what you are doing, so find a way to be accountable so others can get you in the mood to run. There are so many ways to do this. When I first decided to run, I posted on Facebook that I had signed up for a local 5K and would be completing a couch to 5K program. Now, almost 300 people knew of my plans. I had to follow through because I didn't want a single one of them coming to me later and asking about it if I failed. Even if it's just posting a single run, or a planned race, once you have told others that you will be completing it, it gives you more motivation to head out the door.

3. Have the right clothes: If you are only running a mile or two, a cotton shirt and old gym shorts will do. But, if you are going to get serious about running, you need to make sure that you have proper clothes, including dry wicking fabrics, good socks that won't cause blisters, and a decent pair of running shoes. The running shoes are especially important. Without good shoes, you risk injury and discomfort. It's worth investing in them.

If you invest in just one pair of shoes and a couple good outfits, you'll be happy and much more comfortable on the run. Plus, you'll feel more like a real runner if you are dressed appropriately. And if you love it, pretty soon you may end up with more running clothes than daily clothes. It does become an addiction. When you are preparing for your run, make sure you put on your running clothes. Having things you only wear to run helps put you in the mindset of running. Clothes do make the person, after all.

4. Think about how much you hate people who make excuses and do not follow through: We all know the type: they make grand statements about what they want to do, such as write a book, run a marathon, or start their own business. They brag about it all the time. But they never do it! It's all talk and no action. After a while, you get tired of hearing about their future escapades that they never follow through on. The bluster gets annoying. And you don't want to turn into that. So, when you talk about your running, you have to back up your bragging with a little action. If you say you are going to train for a marathon, or even a 5K, back up your words with action. Sign up for the race, do the long training runs, or even find a coach if that's what it takes. Just don't become that person who is all talk and no action. After

all, we all know that that person is the most annoying person in the world.

5. Stop thinking, just go: Instead of debating with yourself about getting out the door, stop thinking about it. One of the tricks to making something a habit is to make one decision and just do it. Instead of arguing with yourself every day whether or not you will go for your run, make the decision that running is non-negotiable. Once that decision has been made, you just go. There is no thinking. There is no worrying about whether it will be good or bad, what the weather is, or if you want to. Like Nike says, Just Do It!

6. Try a different time of day: It can help to keep things interesting. If you normally run in the morning, go for an evening run. If you're used to going out at night, run and watch the sunrise. You may find new inspiration, as the world looks very different at different times of day. This an easy way to mix up your runs without too much difficulty. When you change the time of day, still try to follow the same pre-run routine to get ready.

7. Ditch the tech gear: We all think we need things such as music, running apps, and GPS watches. But, as soon as we rely

on this technology for every single run, we tend to forget the joy of running because we are encumbered by so much junk. To recapture the joy, ditch all the electronics and just go for a run! Remember why you love it. Don't worry about speed or distance, just go and enjoy yourself.

Leave your music at home, dump the GPS, and don't worry about your heart rate. Just run for the sheer fun of it. Remember why you run.

8. Run for charity: Many people want to do something inspiring with their running. You can sign up to run a race for charity and raise money. You could pay for a virtual race that raises money for charity and run on your timetable. You can even dedicate your training runs through an app called Charity Miles. With this app, you turn it on when you run, and corporate sponsors donate money for each mile you run. It serves as a productive way to raise money with all the miles you put in. And you'll feel good that you are putting your time and energy to good use.

9. Get everything ready the night before, making it easier to get out the door: I love to lay out my clothes, get my drink and fuel ready, and have everything sitting out for me in the

morning. That way, I don't have to think. All I need to do is put my clothes on, hit the fridge for a cold drink, and get out the door. I don't have to worry about whether I am missing something, especially when my brain may not be fully awake. It makes it easier, especially when it's early and there seem to be so many other things to do. By having everything at hand, you can just get dressed and go without much thought. This is especially helpful if you aren't a morning person, but are trying to run before work.

10. Dare to be different: Don't copy everyone else. Do something to spice up your training, show off your personality, and have a good time. I have gotten so many comments on some of my running clothes, which are bright and funky. Most people wear boring clothes, usually black. I like tie-dye, paisley, and outer-space prints. I go out of my way to find these things. My favorite site is www.runningfunky.com, although I have begun to find more inspiring clothes in regular stores also. I use running as a vehicle for my personality, and that makes it more fun. I've even had race announcers make comments on these funky outfits as I cross the finish line, which always brings a smile to my face.

11. Have a plan: If you have been winging it, you may not be as consistent as you could be. If you follow a training plan, you have a schedule to run, which can make it easier to get outside. You can get a training schedule for any distance race. They are online, in books, or you can have a custom one made by a running coach or online calculators. Knowing how far you are running each day and when you are supposed to rest can make getting out easier. It takes the guesswork out of training, especially if you have a specific race goal in mind. When you are getting ready for your run, review your plan so you know your goal for the day. Make it a part of your preparation ritual.

12. Leave yesterday behind: We all have bad days. Maybe yesterday's run sucked, or there was some emotional turmoil in your life and you are letting it rule your mind. This is a normal reaction and may make it difficult to get out the door today. However, you cannot let yesterday interfere with today. If you had a bad run yesterday, chalk it up to a bad day. Don't let it deter you from having a good run today. Not all runs can be perfect, but if you focus on the bad, you won't have a chance to make it good. Many people take a single bad run as an omen, causing them to fear the next run.

There have been many times when I have had a terrible, awful run. I was so discouraged because I had difficulty keeping pace for just a couple miles. A few times I have even cut short a longer run because it was so bad. In these situations, I had two choices. The first was to allow myself to become discouraged, dive into the pool of self-hatred, and say I suck at this. That would cause me to give up. The second choice is to say, oh that was a bad day. But I can do better tomorrow. When I say this to myself, yesterday's run isn't that important in the whole scheme of things. And I can get out the door today. It is a new day, after all, and we can rewrite what we think.

Remember, the good runs can only be measured when compared to the bad runs. The bad runs are where character is built, and where you get the choice to decide how you react to them.

Pre-run rituals will help get you into the proper mindset for running. I have found it helpful to have pre-run rituals. When I engage in these activities, my brain knows that it is time for a run and stops protesting. It took me a few months to get to this point, but now, getting out my clothes and dressing while following my other pre-run routines has become part of my warm-up. Next, it's time to hit the road! Plenty of suggestions for hitting the road are described in the next chapter. You should find a few that will help you.

During a run

So many people suffer when in the middle of a run, especially when you are going for longer and longer distances. What many people don't realize is that your mind will quit long before your body needs to. The key to keeping going when the chips are down is to occupy the mind and to encourage it to keep moving. If you can convince your mind that you won't die, your body will continue. In fact, if you can get past that moment of weakness, most people find that they recover pretty quickly and their body actually feels ready to do more than they ever expected. But you can't do that if you don't give yourself a chance to do so. This chapter will give you many tips for dealing with the mind while in the middle of a run.

To me, this is the most crucial aspect of running. I can get out the door, I can do whatever meditations I need while not running, but in the end, what I allow my mind to control while I run will make or break my training. So give these tips a try. You never know which ones will turn into your go-to for gutting it through when things seem to get too tough to go on.

1. Congratulate yourself for putting on your shoes and getting out the doors: Getting dressed and getting out the door is often the hardest part of the run. Once you start, it doesn't seem nearly as difficult. But all the battles in your

mind are subdued when you get out the door. So, congratulate yourself for doing so! You deserve an award for being so committed!

2.   Make yourself run for just ten minutes, then reevaluate: Getting out the door is the hardest part. So, tell yourself that you'll go out for ten minutes, and if you continue to struggle, that you can give up and go home. An odd thing happens with this technique: most likely, you do not give up. Once you are out and moving, it doesn't seem that bad. After your ten minutes are up, you've generally gotten around or close to that one mile point, where your body really starts to get into the workout, and it's not nearly as hard as it you thought it would be. Anticipation is generally much worse than reality.

3.   Imagination: If you are running outside, and it is humid, try imagining a nice, cold, winter day, or a cool fall breeze. Just giving yourself that image can be enough to make a difficult running situation a little easier to take. Imagine the breeze on your back, the coolness of the air, and even breathing freely. When it's hot and humid, this can give you a bit of relief and make it easier to go on through some tough situations. On the other hand, if it's cold, imagine a nice

summer run. It can help warm you up and not think about the snow on the ground (at least for a few minutes).

4.   Runner's math: One of my favorite games is to calculate in my head how much I have run and how much is left to go. For example, I will separate a 15 mile run into three five mile runs, four 5Ks plus 2.6 miles, which is obviously easy since it is shorter than a 5K, or other strange multiples. It's all about breaking up a large task into small ones. It doesn't sound so hard to run a 5K, so I don't need to think about anything but that 5K that I am on. And once I have done 4 5Ks, then, in the last leg, it's only 2.6 miles. My mind can wrap itself around that distance, whereas 15 miles is a distance that it cannot comprehend.

So many people talk about running the mile you're in. This is essentially what this is: breaking up the run into manageable chunks. Many people chunk it even more, only thinking about the mile, or even the half-mile they are currently running. After all, the only thing that we really have is the single moment we are in. Stay in the current mile and don't think about the previous or the next mile.

5.   Find someone to compete with: It doesn't have to be someone who knows you are competing. People I've talked to have imagined racing the person on the treadmill next to them, wanting to go faster or further. On trails, I will try to

keep up with or pass someone who is running close to me. Just knowing that other runners are around me and looking at me is enough to make me want to keep running, even when I am tired.

I also have this weird thing where I don't want other runners to see me walk. This works especially well when I am running on the local trail, where there are many runners going in both directions. If I see a runner coming toward me, it motivates me to keep running even when I want to walk, because, after all, they can't see me walk! Sometimes, it also spurs me to move a little faster than I was before.

6.   Mantras: Affirmations, mantras, and motivational sayings have been used recently for everything from parenting to staying calm. That's because they really work! If you repeat a phrase or word in your mind while you are running, it will help you keep your strength up. I like a three-word phrase, "I am strong," which I will chant in my head, one word for each footfall. After ten or fifteen steps, I have it in my head, and oftentimes, this is enough to keep going, even when I want to stop. I go longer if the first few times don't quite work.

Find a chant or mantra that works for you. Anything that

keeps you going will be adequate. It is helpful if they are short and easy to remember, even when you are struggling. That's why I like "I am strong." I also like "I think I can," from the children's book I mentioned earlier. All that matters is that it is positive, it is easy to remember, and that it motivates you to keep going when you want to give up.

Some good mantras that people use include:

I am strong.

I can. I will.

Fit, fast, fierce.

This will not kill you.

Do or do not. There is no try.

Run hard. Be strong. Don't quit.

Breathe.

Relax and run.

This is fun.

Relentless.

7.   Tune in: If you are in pain, pay attention to that part of the body. For example, if your foot is sore, put all your attention on that foot. Mindfulness meditation practices have shown that paying attention to that area will actually change the pain. You may feel this as you focus your attention on that area. Acknowledge how you feel, notice it, and remind

yourself that pain is only temporary. Just don't stop running (unless, of course, you really have a real injury. Then stop and get help.) You may even notice that your pain changes into something else more tolerable and even find that the pain isn't as bad as you thought it was. I have found great success with this when I get side stitches. It's not a pain that is dangerous, but it can be annoying. By paying attention to it, the pain changes and is more easily tolerated until it goes away.

8.   Tune out: Finding a way to pay attention to anything else but your body works for many people. This is a good reason to run with music (see next tip), have a friend to talk to, or notice your surroundings. Finding a way to forget about the difficulties you go through physically can make the run go much easier. I like to ruminate on a problem or issue that I am having. A run is a good place to clear my head and think differently. And it distracts me at mile 12 of a 15 mile run when I would rather be anywhere else but hitting the pavement.

9.   Music: Music is a wonderful companion on a run. Most runners love to make playlists that empower and energize them. This also gives you something to focus your mind on

when things get tough. Find songs that are encouraging, motivating, and upbeat. I once made the mistake of putting a song on my playlist that I generally found to be funny. It was about a man who lost his girlfriend, and he was talking about all the things they used to do while dating, including eating Twinkies together. It put a smile on my face. But, when I put it on my running playlist, I realized my mistake. The last line of the song, sung over and over, was "I can't go on." This in itself was enough to make me want to quit because, by the time the end of the song hit, where this line was sung over and over, I didn't want to go on either. A more motivating song would have kept me going. So, when planning your playlist, what is on it and what is said in these songs really does make a difference.

There are so many great songs to use. Some of my favorites come from the fact that I grew up in the 1980s, a great time for motivational music. From Survivor's "Eye of the Tiger" to Mathew Walker's "Break My Stride," I find fast beats and motivational messages to be empowering. There are millions of playlist recommendations out there. Google it and see what you find, or just add some songs that you love and that get you moving.

10. Breathing: There are more ways to breathe while running than I can count, so here I will list just a couple that may help you.

First, you can purposely slow down your breathing. You have control over your breath, and you can choose to exercise that fact at any time. If you find yourself breathing heavily, slow it down on purpose. Concentrate on breathing normally. You'll feel less tired if you aren't breathing fast.

Second, try counting your breath. When running, you can count your inhales. Many people will do a count to ten then start over again. This gives you something to focus on when things get difficult. It distracts your mind.

Third, try a controlled breathing method. In the book *Running on Air*, Budd Coates suggests breathing in for three footfalls, and breathing out for two. You can concentrate on how you breathe instead of how you feel when the going gets tough. Similar to mediation, focusing on your breath can help you forget everything else that is going on around you.

11. Mix things up: Do different kinds of training. If you just meander along on the road, try a speed workout on a track.

Hit a trail or try a new route. Your body and mind will function better when you mix up your workouts. You can't run hard all the time or your body will fail you eventually. And you can't always just meander down the road or you'll get bored. Trying different things will keep your workouts exciting.

If you get bored in the middle of the run, you can always do something to mix it up right then and there. One day, I was running and became discouraged because my GPS crapped out. So, instead of worrying about my time, I decided to try a fartlek. A fartlek is the Swedish word for speed play. I would pick a place to run to and speed up until I hit that landmark. For example, I picked out a mailbox about 200 feet ahead of me, then ran with everything I had. When I got to the mailbox, I slowed to a walk. I'd pick another place to run to and do it again, taking breaks in between. It made what I thought would be a frustrating run into something fun and different. It was my first experience of speed work, and I loved it.

By choosing to do a different type of workout, you can really improve your feelings about running. Even mid-run, if you aren't motivated to go on, do something new and different. It will help you go on.

12. Swish on Gatorade, even if you don't swallow it: There is a psychological mechanism at work when you put on Gatorade in your mouth. Basically, your body senses the taste of the drink and assumes it will be getting nourishment, so you start to feel better, even before the drink goes down your throat. You can even spit it out if you don't want to drink it. Just the taste of the Gatorade leads your body to perform better. So, when you start feeling sluggish, take a swig. Me, I like to drink it, but you don't have to. Either way, you should start to feel better almost immediately.

13. Visualize a time that you finished something. Hard. Draw on that strength: We've already talked about visualization while not running, but it can also be an important tool to use while you are running. When things get difficult, you can use visualization during your run. Visualize a time when you had to do something really hard and how you accomplished the task. Visualize yourself finishing strong. You can then transfer that visualization to running. Visualize yourself running strong and finishing well.

If you've had some great runs, visualize those. Bringing back the feeling in your mind of a great run will make a sucky run feel just a little bit better. Visualize when you walked across the stage at graduation, when you finished your first race, or any activity that gave you a rush and a moment of pride. That feeling can be transferred to this specific moment. Knowing that you are strong and capable in other areas of your life will transfer to your running, especially in the moment.

14. Split up your run: Especially on a long run, sometimes it's just difficult to get the entire thing in. Some people do recommend splitting up your long runs. For example, instead of doing a 20 mile run, do two ten mile runs an hour or two apart. Although you don't always want to split your long runs, it is a good strategy once and a while to revive your mind and make it feel more doable.

Just be aware, if you are training for a marathon, it is advisable to do at least one 20 mile run as a single training run, to ensure your body and mind are ready for what it will feel like on race day.

15. Don't be ashamed to walk: This is the hardest thing many runners have a problem with (I know I do). My biggest goal is to get through longer races (half marathon and up) without

any walk breaks. I always feel like walking means that I've failed.

However, truth is that walking is not a failure. It gives you a minute to catch your breath and regroup. Many people find that they can run better and faster after taking a walk break. Plus, walking uses slightly different muscles in the legs, so it gives those muscles a chance to recover. A short break gives you the time you need to tackle round two. And, even if you walk, you are still lapping people on the couch. As long as you are moving forward, it shouldn't matter. Just be sure to get back to running as soon as you catch your breath. It can be too easy to give up and walk every time you feel a little tired. I know each time I do this, it is a little harder to start running again. But a short walk break doesn't give my body time to protest running again. I just make sure I know the difference between being lazy (when I don't want to run) and really needing some time to recover.

16. Think in minutes, not miles: For some people, a mile seems like such a long distance. Their mind seems to work better in minutes. For example, a typical sitcom on TV is 30 minutes (23 if you don't have to watch the commercials). Can you keep going through the time it takes to watch a TV show?

You probably can. So, consider something that takes a certain number of minutes and use that base. Can you run through one sit com? Can you run through two, or an episode of the Walking Dead? Mileage is less important than time on your feet, and may be something easier to wrap your head around.

17. Focus on your body: Your own running style can sabotage your ability to continue. For example, if your body is being held tight and tense, you will be wasting energy on holding your body a certain way. That's less energy available for you to propel yourself forward. This can make it more difficult to finish your run. So, while you are running, you should scan your body to see if you are tense. I find, for example, that I hold a lot of tension in my shoulders. I make a conscious effort to try and relax my shoulders while I run. I try not to hold them too high and instead, allow them to drop, which takes up less energy. Many people hold their fingers in a fist. This also adds tension to the body and wastes energy. Allow your fingers to be loose when running. It may seem like a little thing, but every ounce of energy is valuable as you run longer distances.

Also, if your running form has a lot of extra movements, you will be wasting energy that could be going to power your run.

A lot of people struggle with their arms, and some people allow them to go all over the place. Focus your mind on keeping your arms close to your side, moving back and forth forward. Do not have them cross your body, as this is wasted momentum.

Focusing on your body and your form does two things. First, it gives your mind something to do. Second, it helps make sure your running for is relaxed and efficient, which leaves more energy for what is most important, your run.

18. Make it fun: Remember, running is fun! Think about how it was when you ran as a child. It wasn't for time, it wasn't for exercise. It was for the freedom you felt when the wind blew your hair back and you went as fast or as slow as you wanted. Try to recapture this feeling. Maybe add a skip or a dance. Focus on the music and let it move your body. Enjoy the freedom of movement. After all, what's the point of running if we aren't enjoying what we are doing?

19. Fuel: For any run longer than 60 to 90 minutes, make sure to fuel your body during the run. Your body needs fuel to continue, and having something to eat can serve both physical and psychological benefits. As with the Gatorade

swish described above, as soon as the food hits your taste buds, your body is expecting fuel and performs better, even before it could possibly have utilized any of the fuel you are consuming.

Everyone has their own theories about what to eat in the middle of a run. The easiest thing to do, though not the cheapest idea, is to invest in runner's GU or other foods that are prepared specifically to be eaten mid-run. I've tried a few, but find GU to be disgusting in texture. I've tried some real foods, and found that the thing that gets me through a run the best is Skittles. It has sugar and quick carbs that keep me going and having something that I like really gives me a boost when things are tough.

There are many options for real food, from raisins to pretzels to jelly beans. Experiment and find out what works for you, both physically and mentally.

20. Get out of your comfort zone, then be proud of yourself: Make the run or race more challenging. Sign up for a distance that you've never covered before, do an obstacle or mud race, or experiment with a triathlon (if you can bike and swim, of course). Having a new and unusual challenge will really

spice things up for you. If you keep doing the same thing, you'll get bored and frustrated. Motivation needs to be fueled, and new challenges will do that.

21. Memories of things that motivate you: Think of something that has motivated you in the past, whether it be a person who has run a marathon, a motivational quote, or a movie that you saw that inspired you to train harder. I love thinking of the movie *MacFarlane USA* when I struggle. I'm reminded of the hard life the kids in the movie lived, yet still trained hard for their cross country team. If they could do it, so can I. Specifically, I think of Danny, the kid who struggled the most just to finish, and how he gave all that he had to do so. I can relate to that and can learn from his example. Having some kind of vision such as this really keeps you going.

Some people remind themselves that to be able to run is a privilege. There are people who can't walk, who suffer debilitating injuries, or who have some illness that prevents them from doing what we are doing. Meb, one of my all-time heroes, has talked about his father walking over 200 miles to escape a war-torn country. After that ordeal, running a marathon doesn't seem nearly as difficult.

Whatever you find motivating will work. Just fix that image in your mind when it gets tough. It will give you strength.

22. Imagination: I loved to play basketball as a child. I used to practice on the court at my apartment complex, imagining that I was taking the last shot in a game where we were down by one. If I made it, I would be a hero. If I missed, I would be the goat. Using this same type of imagination will energize your runs. Imagine being in the lead while running an Olympic race, and you can't stop now or you will lose. Imagine the crowd cheering for you. Imagine the people you see on the streets as these fans, your fans are cheering for you and chanting your name. You'll get the adrenaline rush and be want to keep moving so you won't let your fans down.

23. Stay in the now: Mindfulness is a powerful tool. If you are focused only on the present moment, and not what is coming, it is easier to control your body. Many texts, including the books of Jon Kabat-Zinn, espouse the beauty of mindfulness. Check them out.

A simple mindfulness exercise to use when running can be naming your thoughts. Focus only on your environment, how you feel physically and what you see in your immediate environment. If a thought enters your mind, don't dwell on it. Just label it as "thinking." Then go back to focusing on the immediate moment. Notice the way your body feels, the beauty around you, and remember how lucky you are to be able to run and experience this joy. Feel the joy in your body and heart right now. It can be helpful to pay attention to your environment, especially if you run in places that others would find inspiring. One of my favorite runs is going over the world's longest pedestrian bridge, the Walkway over the Hudson. This bridge has been featured in *Runner's World* magazine, and I am lucky enough to live fifteen minutes from it. I often run over the bridge and on the wooded trails it connects. The beauty of the Hudson River, the serenity of the trees, and the peace of not having to dodge cars all contribute to the peacefulness of running. If I'm frustrated, I will notice all these things. I remind myself how lucky I am. I stay in the moment.

24. Brain games: There are so many brain games you can play to distract yourself while running. Remember I Spy? Play it with yourself. Pick a color and look for something of that color. Go over your multiplication tables. Try to remember the states and their capitals. Add random numbers in your head. Anything to exercise your mind and keep it occupied as you run.

25. Reflection: I love to ponder a problem I have when I'm running. The freedom of movement and its repetitive nature is a great time to play things out in my mind and try to find solutions to things that feel like they have no solution. For some reason, when I run, I can see things differently. Use your time running to deal with an issue you have, and you'll get your exercise while being able to look at your issue in a new, and usually more helpful, light.

26. Food/Treat: I met Meb the week after he won the Boston Marathon in 2014. Still reeling from his incredible win, he spent a lot of time talking about how he got through the run and pushed himself to his limit. He told the crowd gathered that he visualized the chocolate milkshake that would be waiting for him at the finish line. We can all take a cue from Meb, especially after a long run. What food or treat will be waiting for you when you finish? Envision that and use it as motivation. I love a chocolate milk after runs over 6 or 7 miles. Envisioning the taste of milk does help me through. Plus, chocolate milk is the perfect recovery drink after a hard workout, so I am not undoing any of my work. For very hard races, especially half marathons and over, I crave meat when I am done running, so I envision the steak that I will get after

the race. The faster I cross the finish line, the faster that steak is in front of me.

27. Pick a spot: This is a very visual way to break up a run. If you get tired, pick a spot in the distance, such as a mailbox, tree, or driveway. Tell yourself that you will run until you hit that spot, then, if you are still having a hard time, you can walk. Once you get to that spot, reevaluate how you feel. If you can still move forward, pick a new spot. I love to play this game because it really does break my run into small, manageable pieces and gives me a spot to focus on. I always know that I can reevaluate how I feel after I hit each specific spot. More often than not, I'm feeling better. I have learned that, the longer I run, as long as the pace is reasonable, the longer I am able to run.

28. Slow down: If you are feeling fatigued, slow down. One common mistake runners make, especially new runners, is feeling the need to run at high speeds. But this is a mistake. Most of your runs should be slow and easy. If you are getting fatigued, slow down. You may not feel like it is running, but it really is. Especially if you are putting in long miles, don't push yourself to go too fast. Your body will never be able to finish the run if you do. If you are out of breath or can't talk for

more than a couple words, you are running too fast. You should be able to hold a simple conversation.

When I first started running, I was lucky if I could run a twelve minute mile. I actually timed myself walking faster than I ran. But the motion of running is different than walking and takes more from your body. If you feel that you have to sprint every time you run, you will wear out far too quickly. Even if it seems silly, slow the pace. It is essential to building you endurance. Speed will come later. Most training manuals recommend running easy runs at 60 to 90 seconds per mile slower than your race pace (especially for longer races such as the half marathon and up). You may not feel that it is doing anything, but running slowly does condition your body.

29. Speed up: Sometimes I have found that running too slowly can be just as draining as running too fast. At this point, I will speed up my run, just a little bit. I have found that focusing on a slow effort can be draining. In these moments, it's important to listen to my body. If speeding up feels good, then I speed up. Sometimes my body is telling me to go faster, that it is ready for it, and that will feel good. Just mixing up the speed will re-energize you.

30. Imagine kicking someone's ass while running: This works well if you're stressed or angry. While you run, think of someone you dislike or are mad at. Use your run to as a stress reliever and envision doing whatever evil things to them that you want to. Fantasy is a great way to get out your frustrations and to motivate you on your run. And by the end of your run, you should feel a whole lot better. Just make sure not to do so in real life.

31. Audiobooks: Instead of listening to music, try getting an audiobook for your phone or iPod. Getting involved in a story, especially on a long run, can make the run more bearable. And you kill two birds with one stone: you get your workout in and you listen to a book on your reading list. Other people will load and listen to podcasts while running. These also keep you occupied while running, and you may learn something new.

32. Take pics of beautiful scenery: Selfies and scenery pictures are motivational, and they also serves as something to post on Facebook after your run. Find a beautiful, inspiring place to run, and take pictures. Enjoy the view. Share what you see with others who aren't as lucky to run as you are.

33. Only turn around at the half way mark: If you always worry that you won't get your miles in, or that you will be tempted to give up early, you could use a trick I have often used for myself, and you'll then only struggle for the first half of the run. If you do an out and back course, you run out for half the distance and then run back. That way, only the first half, when you are fresher, will be a struggle not to turn around. Once you hit the half-way point, you have no choice but to go the entire distance because you are that far from your home or car. When I do smaller bits, I find that it is easier to give up after one loop if I have to do two, or two loops if I have to run three.

34. Get off the treadmill and get outside: Whenever I drive by the gym near my home, I wonder about the people inside on treadmills. I can understand it when it's 10 below, or there's piles of snow on the ground, or there is a thunderstorm, but on a gorgeous spring day, it is much better to run outside. So, if you are a treadmill runner, give it a try. You may dread ever going back to the gym again.

35. Remember, the only person you cheat is yourself: I've seen stories of people cheat by cutting the distance in races to achieve a win or a BQ. However, if you choose to cheat,

even if no one ever finds out, you know that you did not really achieve your goal. You will have to live with that forever. The same is true for every workout. If you cut the run short, the only one you are cheating by doing so is yourself and your goals. If you walk when you're supposed to run, you know it. Remembering that you should not and cannot cheat yourself will help you stay the course.

36. On treadmill, pick a show you will only watch while running: If you do regularly run on a treadmill or are stuck inside because of the weather, make it something special. If you have a show you love to watch, only watch it when you work out. This will motivate you to get to the 'mill cause you want to see what happens next. Knowing that your show is waiting for you can make the dreaded treadmill run easier to stomach.

37. Why are you doing this?: Remind yourself of the reasons you run. Go through the list in your mind. Those reasons should serve a great motivator to you. Write those reasons down. Stick them up on your computer or your bathroom mirror. Keep them close to you at all times. When you need a reminder of why you chose to run, pull them out. Memorize them. This way, when you actually are running, you have the

list embedded in your mind. Going through this list is very motivating when you start to drag. Make sure to memorize this list and go through it on your runs.

38. Remind yourself that if you walk, it will take longer to get done: Walking takes longer, so, if you are trying not to walk, remind yourself that your time will suffer and you will be on the course longer if you walk. Sometimes thinking that this will go on forever is enough motivator to keep you moving. Although walking isn't a sin, I understand the idea of not walking during a particular race or workout. Knowing that I walk a 15 minute mile but run an 11 minute mile can make it easier to run. After all, if I have three more miles to go, do I really want to add on another 12 minutes?

39. Remember how you feel when the run is done: I love the feeling after a run (and after a shower). There is something magnificent about the feeling of satisfaction and accomplishment I get after a run. I glow because I did something hard and did not give up. I feel better because of the endorphins running through my body. By thinking about how happy making my goals makes me, and how I feel so much better after a completed run, I can use this memory to keep me running when the going gets tough.

40. Remember how you feel when you don't run or don't make a goal: It's a negative reinforcement, but it still works. When I give up on a run without a good reason, I feel horrible. I ask myself if I want to feel that way today. Usually the answer is no. Knowing that I hate that feeling is often enough motivation to keep going. Of course, if there is a good reason (such as injury), there is no shame in stopping. But "I don't feel like it," isn't a good reason.

41. Challenge yourself on the course: Make your run more challenging. Increase your speed, try a fartlek, add a hill, or do something else that adds a challenge.

I particularly love the fartlek, which, as I described earlier, is Swedish for speed play. When I run a fartlek, the distances vary and it doesn't matter just how fast I go. This reminds me of running as a child, releasing speed just because I can.

I also do this with hill work. I have a particular route that I run when I want a hilly workout with a large, massive hill at the end. If I want a challenge, this is where I go. And even if I don't make it up the hill all the way, I feel good for having tried. Each time I attempt it, I get a little further up the hill before having to walk. It also helps to see progress.

42. Remember that people pay attention to the good things you do: I like to imagine the people who said I have inspired their running. If I post about a workout or race on Facebook, I don't get a lot of comments. Yet, I have had several people tell me that they have seen my posts or heard me talk about running and that it has inspired them to start. When I want to give up, I think of those people, the people who I know now are paying attention. Knowing that I am doing something good for them, I somehow find more energy to keep going.

With all these suggestions, you will definitely find something that keeps your mind focused during your run, whether you like to tune in or tune out. Either way, trying some of these techniques will help you keep your mind occupied on your run and make them easier. The hardest part of running is to resist the urge to stop. And when that urge hits, there are things you can do! Next, use rewards and post-run rituals to reward yourself for a job well done!

After a Run

After a run, you can keep the positive energy flowing. By using accountability tools, you will feel more motivated to finish the run today and hit the pavement again tomorrow. Try some of these suggestions to make your post-run time more effective.

1.   Accountability: There are so many ways to be accountable for your run. I like to post on Facebook after a run, especially in running groups. There are people there who go through the same things you do and are willing to give you the accountability you need. They give me words of motivation when I am down and pat me on the back when I make a goal. Even a like on a post means someone is paying attention. Another idea is to have a buddy. Even if you cannot run together, you can hold each other accountable for your workouts by contacting each other, such as through texts or emails, when you are done. This way, you always know someone is watching and expecting you to complete your mission. And you don't want to let them down.

If you have an accountability buddy, you could email them your training plan, then, after every run, let them know that you completed it. They can use you for the same thing. If someone is expecting a report, you will be more likely to do the run. Plus, you have someone to brag to!

2.   Don't let a single run get to you. Remember, even the best runners have good days and bad days. If you have a bad day, you must shrug it off, remind yourself that it is only one run, and things will get better. So, instead of spending your after-work out time getting upset because things didn't go well, replay what did go well in your mind, or how you can improve yourself tomorrow. There is always tomorrow, when you can get better. Evaluate what went right and wrong and mentally prepare for tomorrow. Visualization is good for this, as is reminders to yourself that there is something to be learned from every difficult workout. Set yourself up for success.

3.   Pamper yourself off the road: Taking care of your body is a necessity for running, but it can also be a good motivator. For example, after two weeks' worth of workouts, treat yourself to a massage. Done a long run today? Enjoy a luxurious soak in the bathtub, with special bubble bath that you save for this treat. These things feel great, and after hitting the pavement, you deserve them. But, reserve them only for when you do run. If they become part of your everyday routine, they will no longer be a special treat.

4. Gold stars on calendar: Remember being motivated by gold stars as a child? Well, they often work for adults too. After you run, go home and put a star on your calendar. The stars will show how many days a week you have gotten your run in. Putting a star on the calendar and seeing how many days you exercise is a real motivator, especially if you are visually motivated. Put your calendar on the fridge where you, and everyone who lives with or visits you, can see it regularly.

5. Don't watch a TV show till after workout: TV can be a great reward. For example, if you DVRed your favorite show last night, don't watch it until after your run is finished. That will make you want to do it early, so you can enjoy your show without any guilt. Once you've showered and changed, you have earned the right to lay on the couch for an hour or two and watch your favorite shows.

6. Dollar jar: Drop a dollar in a jar every time you work out. Use this money for something special, such as a new workout outfit, GPS watch, or destination race. Knowing your workouts are earning you something you desire keeps you going. And you can watch the dollars add up every day.

Having a post-run ritual and a way to reward yourself will help train your mind and prepare yourself for the run tomorrow. Doing anything that feels good after you run will help you connect those good feelings with completing a workout, which will only serve to enhance the running experience. After all, connecting great feelings to hard work will make you want to do it over and over again.

Conclusion

It is my sincere hope that you found the tips and tricks in this book helpful. Running is as much a mental game as a physical one, and everyone reacts differently to different tricks. Because of this, I tried to vary the techniques described here. Not all of them may work for you, but some of them will. And by following them, you will find the motivation needed to keep running through the hard times as well as the good times.

It's important to note here that runs can be hard, but they can also be great. And, no matter whether your run was good or bad that day, the feeling of finishing it and knowing you accomplished something spectacular (because every run is, in fact, spectacular) is something that you cannot replace. The physical and emotional high of your accomplishments is an experience that cannot be duplicated. And feeling good is what running is all about!

The last thing to remember is that building your mental game can take time. Although many of these techniques can work quickly, to persevere over a long period of time, you need to continue to practice them. Like any muscle, your strength to go forward in the face of difficulty will get better the more you use it. Your mind, just like your body, needs time to train and get better. You won't be able to run a marathon after one day, and your mind won't get stronger with just one or two runs. So keep trying. If something doesn't work the first time, you may have luck with more practice. Or try a different tip. Each run where you win the mental battle will help strengthen your mental muscles, leading to more and more success. You will see changes and improvements, even on days when the run seems too difficult. You can do it!

Happy trails and roads to you!

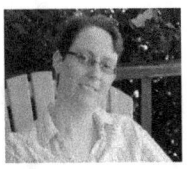

About the Author

Amber Hadigan is a professional freelance writer, singer/songwriter, creativity coach, runner, and a student of the human condition. She obtained her Master's Degree in Transpersonal Psychology from Sophia University in 2004. She was a track rat in school, but stopped running for almost 25 years before taking the sport up again in 2013. Since then, she has devoted herself to becoming the best runner she can be. She has written about her running journey for RunHaven.com and Moonjoggers.com. Amber lives in Hyde Park, NY with her husband John and two cats, Sobe and Scrappy. You can find Amber online at www.amberhadigan.com or email her at amber@amberhadiganwrites.com.